Introduction to Vinegars

Natural Vinegars for Health and Beauty

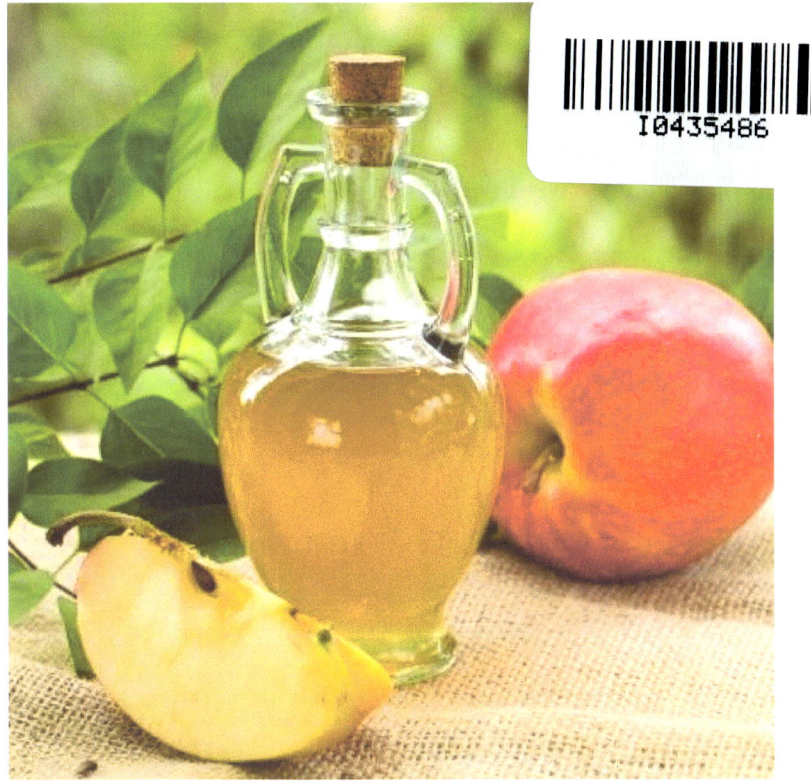

Dueep Jyot Singh

Health Learning Series

Mendon Cottage Books

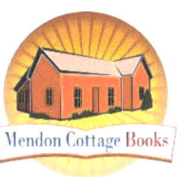

JD-Biz Publishing

All Rights Reserved.

No part of this publication may be reproduced in any form or by any means, including scanning, photocopying, or otherwise without prior written permission from JD-Biz Corp Copyright © 2016

All Images Licensed by Fotolia and 123RF.

Disclaimer

The information is this book is provided for informational purposes only. The information is believed to be accurate as presented based on research by the author.

The author or publisher is not responsible for the use or safety of any procedure or treatment mentioned in this book. The author or publisher is not responsible for errors or omissions that may exist.

Our books are available at

1. Amazon.com
2. Barnes and Noble
3. Itunes
4. Kobo
5. Smashwords
6. Google Play Books

Download Free Books!

http://MendonCottageBooks.com

Table of Contents

Introduction

If you enjoy cooking, or have some interest in herbal remedies, naturally. It is a given that you know all about one of the important ingredients of healing which has been in use for millenniums all over the world in the form of vinegar. Archaeologists have found urns in Egypt, going back to more than 6000 years, with traces of vinegar in them. I would not be surprised if that was just wine which had gone wrong, and somebody decided, all right, we are not going to waste it, we are going to use it for cooking.

The holy Bible refers to vinegar where Ruth was allowed to dip bread in the vinegar – Ruth 2:14-by Boaz. He being an ancient and great wise man would know all about the restorative and healing qualities of vinegar.

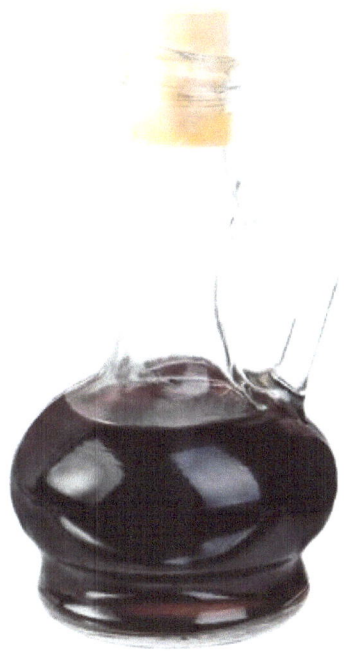

Once upon a time, one of the greatest mischievous activities which I and my brother loved to indulge in was appreciating the homemade orange wine or any other fruit wine made by my father for home consumption, and then smacking our lips, and saying, "Excellent orange vinegar, you have made again dad, where did you go wrong now?"

Of course, the wine was excellent, but it would have him hurrying for a glass of his own, and then wondering what he had done to deserve to such philistines who could not appreciate the difference between good wine and good vinegar. And we would always console him that it would do very well when he was cooking chicken or whatever in a casserole.

Seriously speaking, I can recognize drunk vinegar better than drunk wine, today. In our city's French Institute, they have annual wine and cheese sessions, I was always asked to take the first sip of the open bottle to see whether it was fit for consumption. If I looked at the ceiling pensively, and then wondered whether it was wine I was drinking, the bottle would be finished immediately. But the moment I said "oh wow, what is this stuff", – only those desperate enough to finish the bottles would drink from that particular bottle. It took me 3 years to find out that I was the official vinegar tester!

Naturally, in ancient times, vinegar, which has a large percentage of acetic acid, was not only used for healing and for beauty purposes, but it was also used to give dishes a sour taste.

Let me tell you another amusing story. My French cordon bleu cook friend, François, was making up something tasty for his guests, and family one leisurely weekend, and he just happened to say, where is the wine? I busy poking my nose in the kitchen, along with him and getting in his way asked him whether acetic acid would do instead?

I really loved to wind him up while his wife, Dominique, and his children and grandchildren listened to him lose his cool, and splutter and yell "Aceetic" acid, and you call yourself ze Cuhk."

According to him, any person substituting acetic acid for wine vinegar, was capable of substituting tinned tomatoes or sun-dried tomatoes for homemade tomato sauce, and sandwich spread in salads instead of real homemade mayonnaise. What about the subtle overtones of flavor, what about the glowing rich color, what about the finished dish's rich fragrant aroma, and so on and so forth. Until he would look up and see a whole admiring throng of guests, grinning 3 deep in the sidelines.

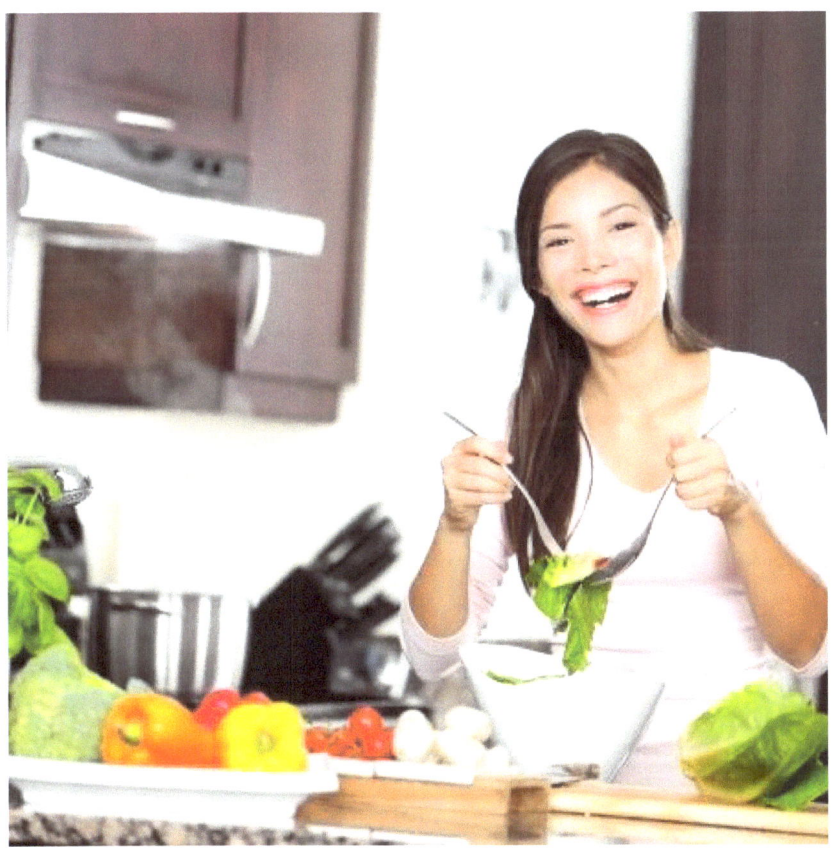

In medieval times, they tell about the black plague tormenting Europe where people were so desperate to save themselves that they left their doors open and ran away, not bothering much about their belongings. However, there were 4 crafty thieves, who could not be bothered about any sort of infection because they had made up a mixture told to them by an old witch – how did she prevent herself from getting burned at the stake – and this is what the recipe says.

Take 1 L of cider vinegar; add 3 teaspoons full of crushed garlic to it, and 2 teaspoons each of dried peppermint, rosemary, and sage. To this add 1 teaspoon each of nutmeg, ground cloves, and cinnamon.

This is the greatest antiseptic you could ever find when you put all the ingredients in a blast vessel and allowed to stand in strong sunlight for 15 days. Strain and bottle, and whenever you are going in an infectious area, do what the 4 thieves did, cover your face and your hands with clothes dipped in this mixture, and you are not going to get infected. Also, cover your feet, if you are robbing the dead on the streets.

Well, they supposedly plea bargained for freedom, by giving their judges this recipe, but knowing about those ruthless times, I am hundred percent sure that they were dispatched yea verily, foresooth and right speedily by the ruthless judges so that they could not go around telling everybody else about this cure.

Vin aigre is the French word for sour wine, hence where the word vinegar comes from. This term is also used when referring to alcohol-based liquids that are sour since they are made with malt, cider, or rice wine.

Making of Vinegar

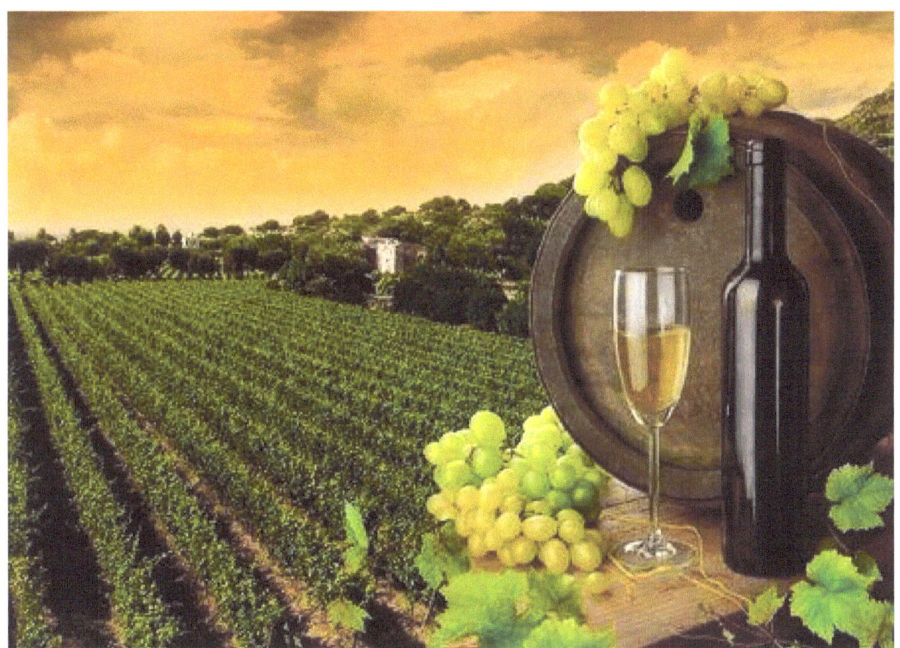

Just like wine, good vinegar is also going to be made in casks.

This souring is, of course, a natural process that happens when liquids with less than 18% alcohol come in contact with the air.

A reaction occurs when the bacteria in the air comes in contact with the alcohol, it makes a thick, moldy looking skin the covers the surface of the liquid. This is known as the "mother liquid," which is basically a layer of yeast, which makes a natural acid out of the alcohol. The acid is what is going to give the vinegar its distinct flavor.

Although this reaction is going to occur naturally, it's not always consistent, because there are a number of factors which are going to either delay or promote this fermentation process. To produce high quality vinegars the speed and the temperature of this process has to be monitored, regulated, and controlled. In ancient times, people were experienced enough to know exactly when the vinegars could be taken out from the casks, but today winemakers and vinegar makers have a completely scientifically controlled process used in making wines.

But now you are going to say, if you leave an open bottle of wine exposed to the air, could return into vinegar, because after all, there is going to be some fermentation going on somewhere. Alas and alack, that is not going to happen. Otherwise, we would all be having plenty of wine vinegar, ready at hand.

So due to this temperature and the speed process, we are going to have delicious tasting vinegar, but if it is unmonitored, we are going to have lots of flavor, and also bitter flavors, when the bacteria are allowed to proliferate uncontrolled.

Sushi is not complete without rice wine – sake – and wine vinegars are essential in salad dressings and marinades.

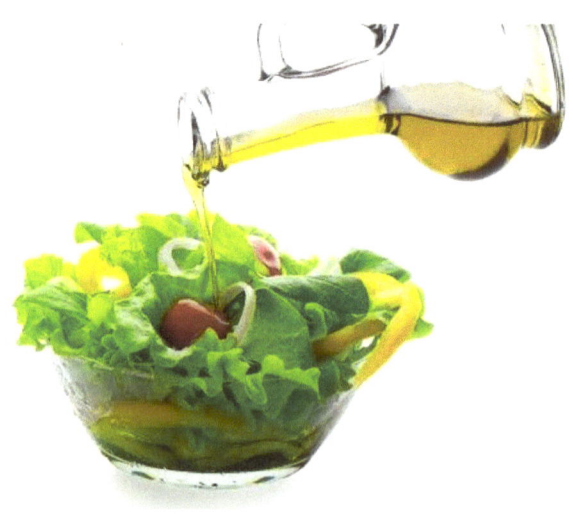

And if you are in Britain and dining off fish and chips, you cannot do without malt vinegar on them, which are incidentally also going to be making up the authentic traditional pickles, and also the traditional British piccalilli[1]. Vinegar used to make pickles is going to preserve the vitamins and minerals of the fresh vegetables and also promote the digestion while the spices are going to add simulative and healing warmth to the mixture.

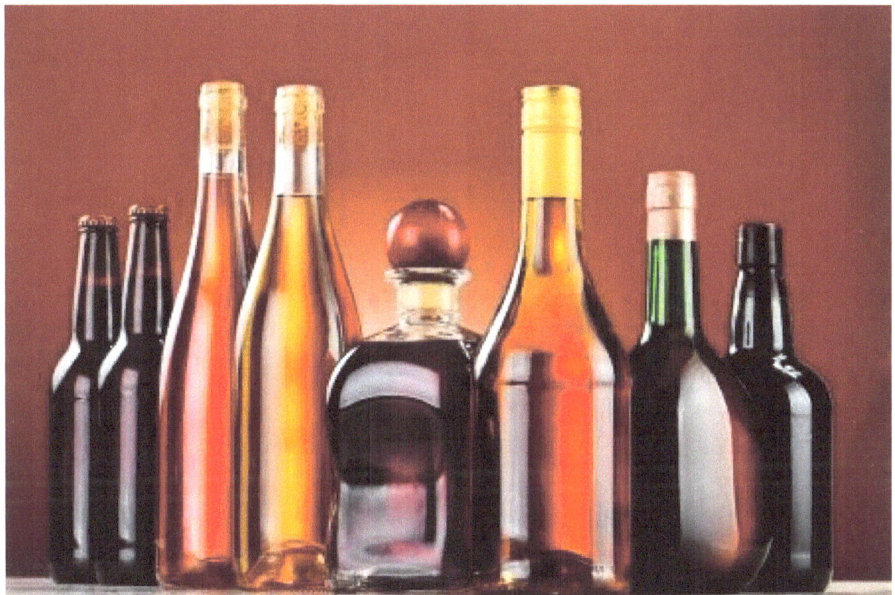

---

[1] There is an amusing story about how this particular dish got its English name. When India was part of the British colonies, a Saheb with a business turn of mind , somewhere in the eighteenth century, was exploring the markets to find out which spices to export, when he happened to look at the pickles spread out before his eyes in a local shop. "my word, pickles", he exclaimed, and the shopkeeper nodded his head wisely, and said, "yes, yes, Sahib, piccallilli." And so the Britisher thought that that was the word used in the local vernacular to describe that highly spiced traditionally made aromatic condiment known all over the world as "pickles."

You can make vinegar from wine, Sherry, cider, rice, and malt. In most cases, wine vinegars normally required at least 6% of acetic acid and other vinegars are going to range between 4 – 6% acetic acid. The slight variation in the acidity level is going to be of concern, when you are preparing preserves and pickles, especially when they are only barely noticeable to the taste. However, a very high acidic level is going to make you make faces all over the place and wonder whether it is polite to spit out those terrible pickles in public. [Not polite. You just put a paper napkin to your mouth and spit it out in that! Then crumple the paper napkin into the nearest dustbin.]

Strong vinegars can be made from wine, malt, and cider; the strongest flavors come from spirit and distilled vinegars. Malt vinegar is the most commonly used for distilling, even though any vinegar can be distilled. Through the process of distilling, the acetic acid level is brought to more than 6%.

If you were traveling all over the world, you are going to see that the vinegar made in that particular country is going to depend upon the produce. For example, winemaking countries like France, Spain, and Italy are going to produce wine vinegars.

On the other hand, in the Middle East, where wine is not made often due to cultural and other traditional reasons, vinegars are normally made up of dried raisins. Where apples are in abundance, like in the United States, you are going to get Apple cider vinegar. In Japan, you are going to get rice wine, turned into rice vinegar. This just has about 2 – 5% of acidic acid and is comparatively mild. Beer brewing countries like Germany and Britain are going to produce malt vinegar.

Wine Vinegar

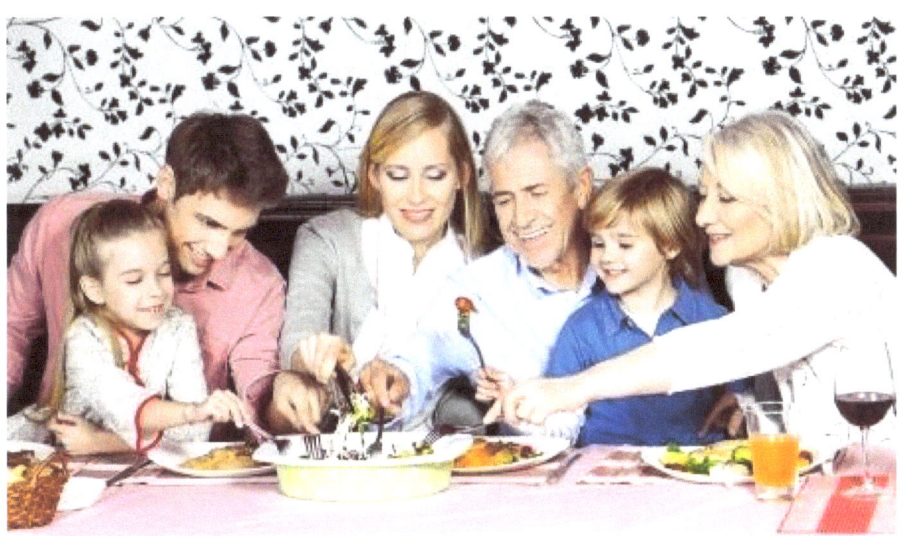

A little bit of wine helps in the celebration, and is also healthy, so is wine vinegar.

This is produced from both red and white wines and the quality of the vinegar is going to depend on the quality of the wine. The finest wine vinegars are made by the Orleans method which is going to allow the wine to ferment slowly and naturally at about 70°F or 21°C in oak barrels until the mother forms on the surface.. However, this was the traditional way in which wine was made when people had plenty of time and leisure to make wine and also vinegar, and comparatively, it is costlier now to make this particular wine vinegar. And that is why manufacturers, in the 21st-century, look for quick ways of speeding up the fermenting process. This is done by raising the temperature. This is going to result in a less costly vinegar but of course, the quality is going to deteriorate proportionately.

There are almost as many types of vinegars made out of wine, as there are wines in existence. That means you are going to have a champagne vinegar which is of a pale color and delicate in flavor. A Rioja vinegar made in Spain is going to have a deep red color, and a full, rich taste. A sherry vinegar is very popular used extensively in cooking because of its deep caramel color and find rich, mellow flavor. This is normally matured in wooden casks, similar to those, which are used in the making of Sherry and that is why it is comparatively expensive to make this particular Sherry vinegar.

As Australia and the United States are developing more wines for public consumption and for profit, new kinds of vinegar, especially California Zinfandel grape vinegar varieties are emerging and getting to be really popular.

Balsamic Vinegar

There is one particular wine vinegar that is gaining recognition in cuisines all over the world. We know it as balsamic vinegar, originating in a small town in northern Italy called Modena. When I first heard of it, my mind immediately associated it with the balsam flower, but actually it is the Italian word for Balm. This means that it has a smooth mellow character.

Balsamic vinegar is normally made from unfermented grape juice that is aged in wooden casks. The quality of the finished product is going to depend a great deal on the type of the wood which has been used and the skill of the vinegar maker.

The finest vinegars are aged for a minimum of 10 years! Just imagine anybody having this much patience in today's world, where you do not know what is going to happen at the next moment and time is working at hyper speed and there is no time to stop and stare! That is the reason why balsamic vinegar needs experience, artistry, and all the care taken, which is used in the production of a great wine. So the next time you are in Modena you may find yourself drinking this wine vinegar as an after dinner drink.

Traditionally made original balsamic vinegar is quite expensive. However, you can get industrially made substitutes and versions, and these are the acceptable substitutes which are being used in cuisine, in most traditional recipes.

This aromatic vinegar was originally made with white grapes and allow to rest in casks made up of Chestnut, mulberry, juniper, cherry, ash wood, and oak. Naturally, it took anywhere between 10 to 25 years to get the final product and that is why only the Italian aristocrats could afford this vinegar. The form which you are going to get in the market today is called balsamic vinegar made up of any sort of grape juice in which you have mixed some vinegar, colored with a caramel color and sweetened with sugar, caramel, and grape juice concentrate. This is the twentieth century product being sold as original balsamic vinegar – but it is definitely not that.

Balsamic Vinegar Made at Home

Anyway, here is the recipe for balsamic vinegar, made at home and it is spiced but not cured for 25 years in casks. For this you are going to need 6 cardamom pods, 12 black peppercorns, 12 golden raisins, one teaspoonful of rosemary, one teaspoonful of sage leaves, 4 cloves, and 1 ¼ cup of cider vinegar.

Crush all the ingredients together, and allow to seep in the vinegar for about 2 months in the sun. Then strain and bottle. Traditional balsamic vinegar is going to have a number of other herbs and spices, depending on the availability and the time, but you can always experiment with your own combinations of spices and herbs.

After all, you want a vinegar, which is a good medicine, giving you nourishment. You can use this vinegar either in cooking or as a salad dressing. To use as a drink or a stimulant, tonic, or a balancer, skin wash or a cooler, compress, or a cooling lotion or hair rinse, you are going to dilute one tablespoonful of this vinegar in 1 cup of hot or cold water.

Cider Vinegar

Apple pulp or cider can be made into cider vinegar following the same method which you use to produce wine vinegar. There are recipes that call for special traditionally made cider vinegar, but it has a sharp and a strong flavor and should be used when it complements the other ingredients. Commercial cider vinegar is filtered and is a pale brown substitute. Homemade cider vinegar can become cloudy but this does not affect their taste or indicate that the quality is inferior. The flavor is not smooth, and that is why it is restricted only for salad dressings. However, you can use it for making fruit pickles successfully.

How to Make Cider Vinegar.

In herbal medicine wine insider vinegars are naturally favored for their gentle action. To obtain all the trace elements with vitamins, trace elements and flavor, vinegar is normally made from a vinegar Mother. Traditionally, these mother recipes were passed down from generation to generation, and every grandmother knew about her particular cider vinegar recipe, which would stay in the family. Many European villages made vinegars as distinctive as the local wines available for home consumption.

One-sided, vinegar culture can be maintained and fed in a wide mouthed traditional earthenware crock. Contamination is prevented by using scrupulously clean utensils.

So we are going to be making cider vinegar with as many apples as we can get because we are going to utilize the waste Apple peel and cores and enough water to cover. Scrub the apples scrupulously in plenty of water. There is plenty of nutritional good stuff just below the peel, but make sure that the peels do not have any sort of pesticides or chemicals sticking to them. That means, if you get organic apples, so much the better.

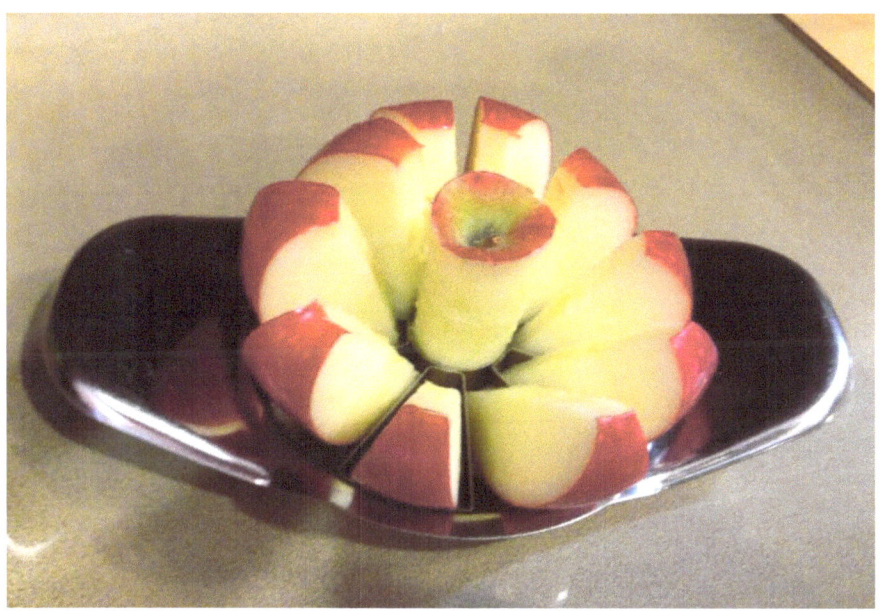

Peel and core the apples. All types of apples are suitable, but it is preferable that you use just one variety as you are going to get slightly different flavor to the vinegar. For example, you may use Granny Smith and Cox Sweet for different types of vinegars. Bramley's are going to give you an invigorating and clear vinegar.

Use as many flesh apples as you want. Put the Apple peel and the cores in a wide mouthed earthenware crock and just covered with pure water. Cover the crock and put in a warm place and allow it to ferment.

This recipe is going to work best with the core and peels of at least 12 apples in the beginning. If you are using much less than this, add half a cup of apple juice. This means that you are going to use less water to cover.

Taste the liquid every few days and stir so that the air may continue the fermentation process. Remove the froth as it ferments. The taste of the vinegar is going to develop gradually depending on the temperature and the cloudiness of the liquid is going to clear slowly.

When it is to your taste, it is ready to strain into a large bowl. Empty the crock in preparation for the next batch. You may need to rinse it with water, or you can just wipe it but never use any sort of detergent or soap for cleaning purposes. To make a fresh batch, you are going to add fresh apple peels and cores. Add vinegar mother and enough water to cover. Repeat the steps again until you have your preferred cider vinegar.

Pour the majority of the vinegar into a bottle and label it with the date of manufacture and bottling. Once the vinegar has reached its full vinegar taste, there is no more alcohol to ferment and it is going to become a stabilized product when it is bottled. The vinegar should not deteriorate from then on.

Return a small amount of the vinegar to the crock to become the vinegar mother for future vinegars.

To keep the vinegar mother healthy and alive, until you next wish to make some more apple vinegar, just add peel and water occasionally to the liquid left in the crock.

Quick Wine Vinegar

One bottle of your favorite red or white wine or sherry dry and one tablespoonful of pot barley.

This is the traditional way in which you can make quick Wine vinegar by putting the wine or the sherry in a earthenware crock and adding the barley. Allow it to stand in a warm place for a few days.

When you think it tastes just right, which is going to be about 2 or 3 days, strain, bottle, and label. Keep some of the liquid and return it to the crock. This is going to become your starter or mother liquid. In ancient times, this mother was maintained and kept alive by feeding her occasionally with the dregs of fine wine. Always use the same type of wine, red or white to keep "mother" healthy.

Malt Vinegar

If you are living in an area where malt beer is drank in large quantities, it is natural that you are going to have local malt vinegar which is made traditionally of malted barley. This is often used as a pickling vinegar because it has a very strong flavor and is not very good for salad dressing, however, it is good for pickling vegetables like onions and other which are sharply flavored. Cucumbers and other watery vegetables are pickled excellently in malt and also, chutneys and sauces are complemented properly with a malt vinegar base.

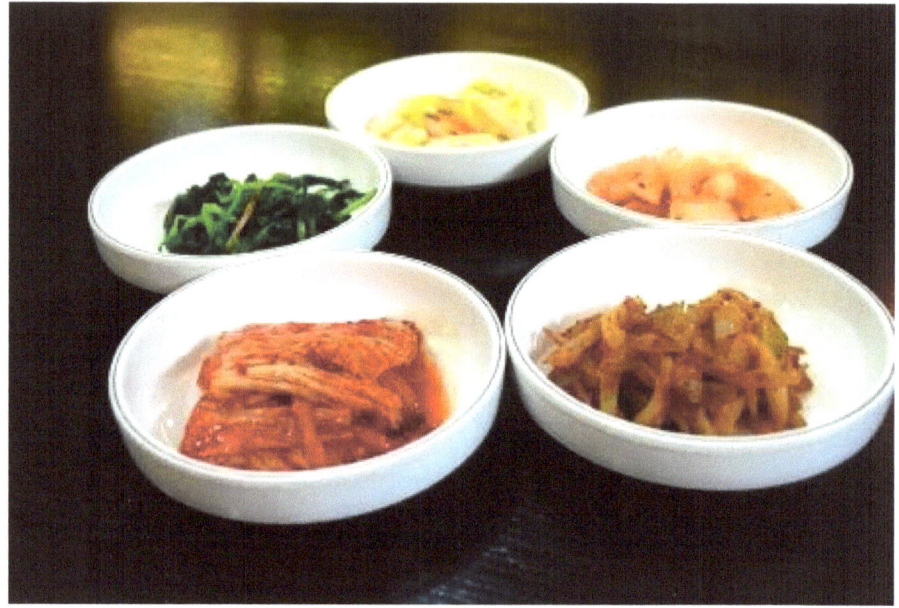

Spirit Vinegar

This vinegar is the strongest of all the vinegar types and varieties. And that is why it is used for exclusive pickling purposes,. The only difference between this particular vinegar and distilled vinegar is that it is going to have a little quantity of alcohol in it.

Rice Vinegar

If you have ever lived in the East, especially in China, Japan, and Thailand, you may have appreciated the cuisine in which rice vinegar is used extensively. This type of vinegar is going to be made of fermented and soured rice wines. Wine vinegar in Japan is going to be mild and mellow, but the Chinese variety is going to be slightly sour and sharp in taste. Depending on the rice used, Chinese vinegars are normally white or red in color. Sometimes it is also flavored. Sweet rice wine known as mirin and soy sauce is also added to this rice vinegar along with spices and flavors like horseradish, mustard, chilies, gingerroot, and even flakes of dried fish. They use so many spices, because the end product is going to be used extensively in cooking to impart a subtle flavor to the dish.

In China, you can also find black Chinese vinegar, which is made up of millets, sorghum, and wheat instead of rice. So make sure that your vinegars are stored away in a cold, dark place, no refrigeration is required. If stored correctly, most vinegar can keep for an indefinite period of time.

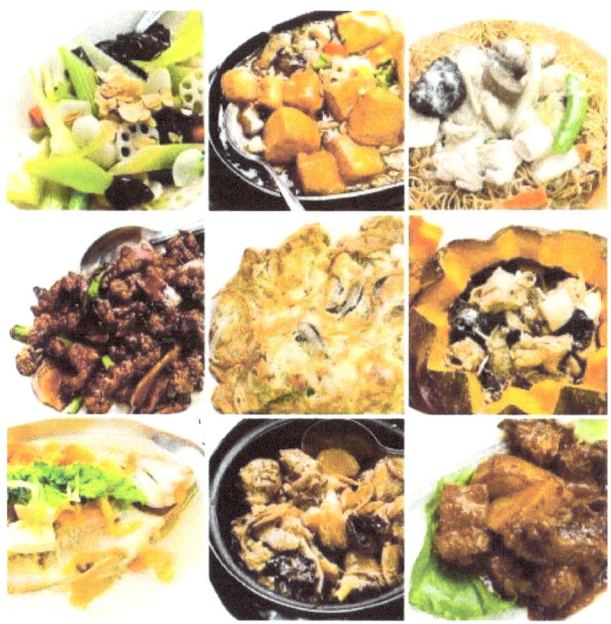

Eastern cuisine is going to have a touch of vinegar in it, without fail.

Vinegar in Cuisine

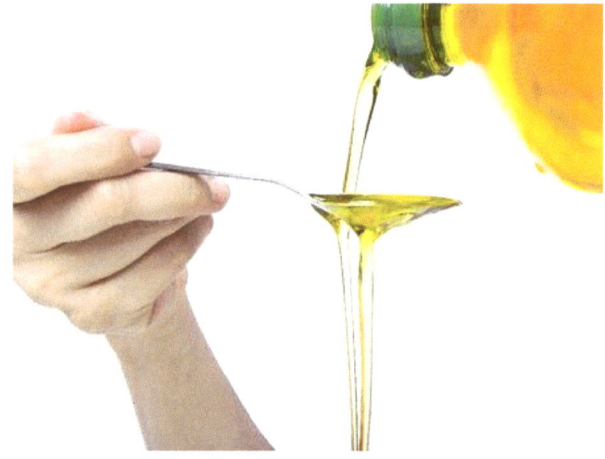

The importance of a really good vinegar, which is used to flavor a finished dish can never be overlooked. Unfortunately, we do not bother much about the flavor of flavored Chinese vinegar or a touch of balsamic which has been made of the best ingredients to transform an ordinary dish into something fit for a Chinese Emperor or the Czar of Russia.

Certain kinds of vinegar are used to "deglaze" juices in the pan, for strong sauces or for gravies. Adding some vinegar can enhance many sauces especially those whose base is tomatoes, but remember a little goes a long way. Too much vinegar is going to spoil the broth just like too many cooks. Try a little bit of vinegar with raspberries and strawberries as well as fresh fruit salad, especially if the vinegar is mellow and gentle.

For example, if you are eating out in Modena and are enjoying the traditional fare, it is possible that you are going to be offered sliced strawberries and balsamic vinegar. This is made by drizzling fresh strawberries with high quality balsamic vinegar and allowed to mellow for half an hour before serving. In the same manner, a few drops of balsamic vinegar is used, to deglaze pan fried duck or liver and make a really delicious flavorsome dish.

Choosing the Right Vinegar

When you are deciding upon the vinegar to use in a particular dish, if the recipe calls for a vinegar and it has not told you which particular variety – I have seen many French and Italian recipes calling for balsamic vinegar, but other recipes say, 1 teaspoon vinegar – always choose a vinegar with a complimenting flavor. Malt vinegar has a strong flavor, since it is made from grain, it goes best with solid foods, such as cold meats, relishes, chutneys, or fish and chips.

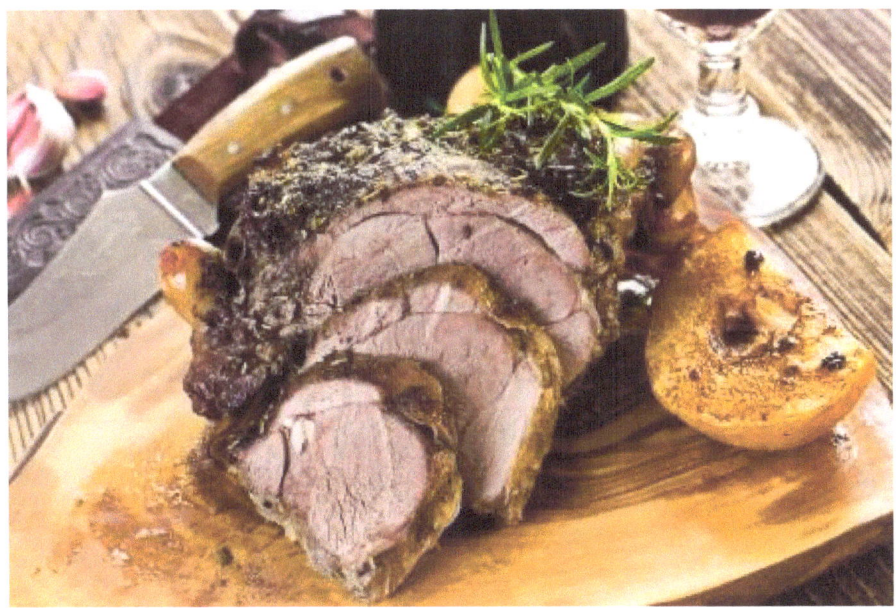

A little bit of malt or balsamic vinegar would make a great compliment

On the other hand, cider vinegar is the best choice when you are deglazing pork chops accompanied by sautéed apples. Incidentally, pork goes very well with apples and that is why one of the greatest and very often used unoriginal literal clichés in fiction is the statement of "I would not have him if you served him up to me on a silver platter with an apple in his mouth." Traditionally, hogs heads and roasted boar were served at wedding feasts in this manner, especially the silver platter and the head glazed with honey.

Deglazing is a cooking technique, where first the baked or fried dishes are removed from the pan for either resting before serving or baking. You are now going to add some wine, water, stock, or any other liquid to this hot baking dish or frying pan, in which you were cooking the meat previously. The browned residue remaining at the bottom of the pan is scraped off with the liquid and stirred so that all the browned delicious bits have been molten into the wine, vinegar, or water on a moderately high heat and then poured over the meat, if it is still baking or you just want a delicious gravy.

When you are making mayonnaise and any type of salad dressing, wine vinegars are best suited. They are excellent for making a number of butter based sauces such as béarnaise, which was originally made with white wine vinegar and served with fish. – a fine wine vinegar is also going to add distinction to a rich meat dish or a game stew.

Using Vinegar for Herbal Infusions

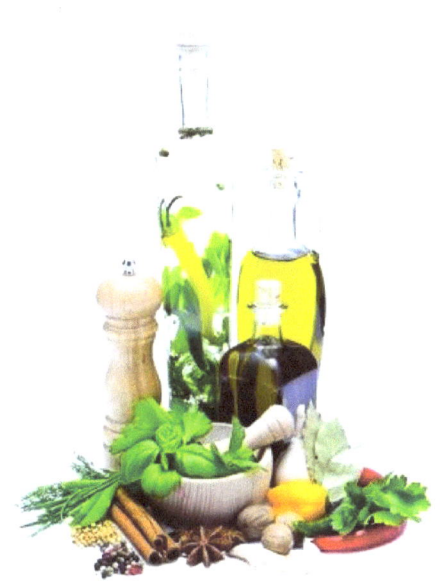

In ancient times, dried herbs were stored in tight pottery jars or in dark glass jars. Clear glass containers were stored inside kitchen cabinets and in sellers. That was because light and exposure to the air and moisture made the herbs deteriorate more quickly. And this is the reason why it is important to make sure that all the containers are well sealed, before you keep them in a dark place.

Freezing is another effective way in which you can extend the availability of the herbs, especially basil, fennel, parsley, and dill. This is done by cleaning the herbs as appropriate and sealing in small quantities about 2 – 3 tablespoons, in freezer bags. You can either freeze them, alone or in your favorite combinations. You can also make them into a tomato sauce seasoning with thyme, basil, oregano, and parsley. Use a large strong container for all the herbal bags, before you freeze them, which means that you do not have to empty out the refrigerator freezer in order to get frozen herbs. It is also going to protect them from damage.

I often use ice cube trays to make individual herb cubes. This is done by scissoring the herbs really finely, half fill each ice cube compartment with the chopped herb and fill the rest with water. Freeze. Then remove the cubes and put them in your favorite freezer bags for easy access.

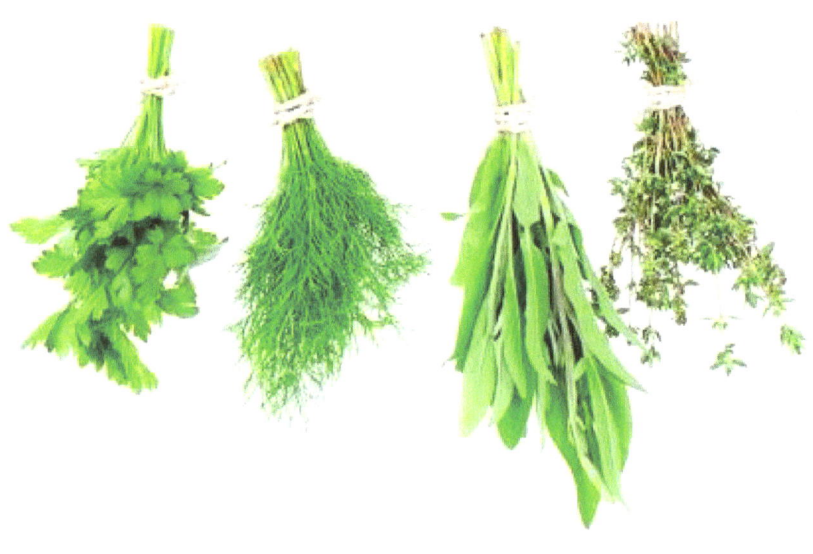

Naturally, the traditional way in which the herbs were infused and preserved was by bruising the herbs lightly and then placing them in a large glass jar. After that, warm vinegar was poured over them. Good quality wine and Sherry vinegars work best for this particular purpose. Do not use a metal container, just because it is so easily available in the 21st-century! Untreated aluminum is going to work adversely, when it comes in contact with vinegar, as well as leaving a metallic taste to the end product.

Use light-colored vinegar so that you can see the herbs through them.

You can leave it to infuse in the sun for about 3 weeks stirring daily. Taste at the end of the infusion time. If it is not strong enough for your taste, discard the herbs, and add more fresh herbs then leave for another week or so.

Strain the vinegar to remove any vestiges of herbs. If desired, you can transfer to any sort of decorative bottle and a fresh sprig of the herb for decoration purposes and so that you can recognize the vinegar at first sight.

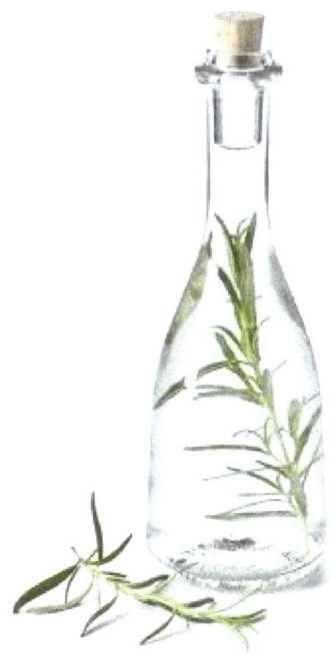

Use only seals and caps which have plastic linings for vinegar. If you can get old vinegar bottles, this is going to be the perfect choice, especially when their caps are all made to measure. Here are some excellent traditional vinegar and herb combinations – cider vinegar with applemint, white wine vinegar with tarragon and thyme, and red wine vinegar with rosemary and garlic.

Here is another way in which you can preserve your favorite herbs like basil. Just place the whole leaves in your blender after washing and cleaning thoroughly with a few teaspoons full of lemon juice, a few cloves of garlic, and just enough of olive oil/vinegar to cover. Process until all of them are mixed thoroughly. Transfer to a clean jar with air tight covers then refrigerate or freeze in ice cube trays.

Incidentally, pure Apple cider vinegar is going to need a little bit of dilution with fruit juice, or with honey if you are using it as a health enhancing drink.

Fruit Vinegar

Incidentally, fruit, especially strawberries and other berries can make a delicious vinegar just by covering the fruit with vinegar and leaving it to stand for 2 weeks and then straining and bottling the liquid.

Fruit vinegars are best made when you have plenty of soft fruit and berries so that the minerals and the vitamins are preserved for use, especially during the cold dark winter.

In winter, you are going to take 1 teaspoon in a cup of water or according to your taste. Fruit vinegar is cleansing and sharpening especially when you take it first thing in the morning. This is your wake-up tonic for your whole system, and to prevent or ease colds, coughs, and fevers. Also, iced fruit vinegar is excellent and cooling, especially when you are using it on a hot summer day.

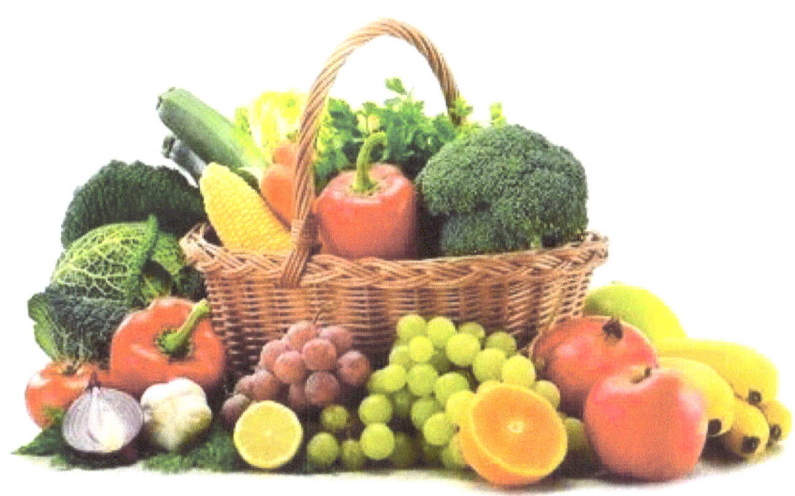

Any soft fruit can be used, to make fruit vinegar.

Also, this particular tonic is excellent, first thing in the morning if you are suffering from rheumatism and arthritis. That is because of its antiseptic qualities. You can also use this as a bath for thrush conditions and personal hygiene. Also, if you are suffering from fungal infections like athlete's foot, this is going to get rid of that problem while preventing any sort of further trouble. Just apply vinegar straight on the affected area.

Spicy Vinegar

Any sort of vinegar which has been flavored with herbs and spices is going to make an excellent flavoring addition, when added to your cooking and salad dressing. You can also use them for cool and refreshing drinks, hair rinses, and skin lotions.

In our area, traditional vinegar is made up of sugarcane, of which you are going to add the juice to an earthenware crock with real honest-to-goodness traditional hundred percent iron nails! Nothing else is added to it, and the fermentation is going to occur due to the sugarcane and the yeast in it. It is excellent for adding just this bit of stronger flavor to pickles, meats, and for flavoring hot and spicy curries.

What Is Distilled Vinegar?

When I saw this product in the market for the first time, it was a state of "Duh?" I knew it was a commercially made product, especially when it is used as a cleansing product made from petroleum. Actually, this is not any sort of distillation being done to the vinegar or its original source, but more of fermenting alcohol, which has been distilled. This is going to have about 8% acidic acid content with a pH value of 2 . 5. This is also known as white vinegar, lab vinegar and also distilled spirit, especially when you are using it for scientific research purposes, medicinal, and lab purposes.

I remember us at university, yelling for the distilled spirit, in our Chemistry, Botany, and Zoology research practical labs, supposedly for finishing an experiment, but more for dabbing on your hand and taking a hearty sniff to see how long it took for the alcohol to cool the skin. Spirit meant alcohol in any form and sniffing alcohol during class hours give us a vicarious crazy man, far out sort of loony thrill. Nothing came out of it, but it was a good way to waste time! This was the spirit/spirit vinegar – which I later used, to get rid of all the varnish on my wooden furniture before the re – varnishing and re-polishing to a high gloss.

Incidentally, white vinegar is what is normally used for preserving meat, especially when you do not have the original stuff with you, and also for pickling. Malt is the best starter for this particular vinegar, in many regions where malt is easily available and because of the low cost. The Heinz distilled vinegar brand is made up of corn. Malt vinegar is also known as alegar.

If you are visiting Japan and you find Kurozu being sold there as a health promoting drink, it is black vinegar, traditionally made from rice. The ancients made sure that they never suffered from any sort of health problems including cancer, by drinking diluted Kurozu or using it often in their cuisine. Thanks to its high amino acid content and concentration, it is good for your basic general health. Also, the salad dressings in Japan and the sushi are going to be flavored with rice vinegar. Because it may have a mild sort of flavor, it is seasoned with herbs and spices beforehand to give it a stronger flavor and kick.

Vinegar for Good Health

In ancient Greece, a vinegar was made up of honey mixed with vinegar called oxymel. Nowadays, researchers are looking at the benefits obtained from original oxymel, which incidentally was used as a health giving beverage and a medicine in ancient and medieval Europe.

When I first tasted the traditional Persian shekanjabin, I remembered that the name had the same sort of origins as a traditional drink in our area called shekanjvi, made up of lemons, mint, honey, and water and then boiled to make a syrup. This concentrated drink was then drunk 2 spoons to a glassful of water with ice, especially when we were totally dehydrated. This particular Persian drink was made up of fruity vinegar, in which honey water or sugar water was added and then drank. Well, lemon juice and honey water or fruity vinegar, water, and honey, everything traditional is going to be beneficial.

Incidentally, if you eat salads made up of pure vinegar and oil dressings often, there is less chances of you suffering from heart diseases. I do need to be a researcher to tell you this. Your salad is going to have plenty of fresh fruit and vegetables in it. Why waste so much money in researching something which is evident, and concentrating on vinegar as a dressing, when everybody knows that it has kept the heart healthy for millenniums, and through different cultures? Also down the ages, teas which were made of vinegar were used, to control diabetic symptoms when about 25 g of natural vinegar was added to the meals and fed to the patient. It is also good for non-diabetics.

In Regency times, Lord Byron started up a new fad in order to keep his weight under control. Whenever he went out in a social gathering, he asked for biscuits and vinegar. Actually, about 700 mg of acetic acid taken in any form is quite capable of reducing obesity because it makes you feel less hungry. But then, his grateful hostesses never knew that right after that social function, he would go straight off to one of the Prince of Wales' regular parties and have anywhere between 6 to 12 courses for drinks and dinner. He was dangerously overweight, and used a corset to keep his full figure within control, but that did not stop him from eating, drinking, and living it up Regent Size.

I remember getting really badly cut in one of my too frequent accidents in the kitchen, and not finding any antiseptic anywhere ready at hand, I just took out some vinegar and some honey, applied it all over the cut and allowed it to dry in the air without bandaging it. Later on I found out that the ancient Egyptians and Babylonians used vinegar for getting rid of any possible infections – external and internal. They also used it for curing fevers, constipation – 2 tablespoons vinegar in a glassful of water – and so on. People are now researching on how vinegar can cure tuberculosis, but believe it or not, this was done in ancient Babylon with the patient put on a meat diet, with plenty of vinegar in it, along with a highly proteinaceous diet, along with dry fruits, spices, and lots of honey on the bread with fresh butter and buttermilk.

If there is anyone among you who does not believe in modern medicines and somehow have managed to fall prey to tuberculosis or any other respiratory disease, you may want to try out this highly effective ancient traditional medicine recipe given above. Remember that the vinegar has to be pure and not the distilled sort masquerading as vinegar. May the ancient gods of health be with you. Also remember that the spices and herbs you are going to use are going to be cinnamon, garlic, ginger, cloves, cardamoms, onions, lots of peppercorns, and, of course, lots of honey.

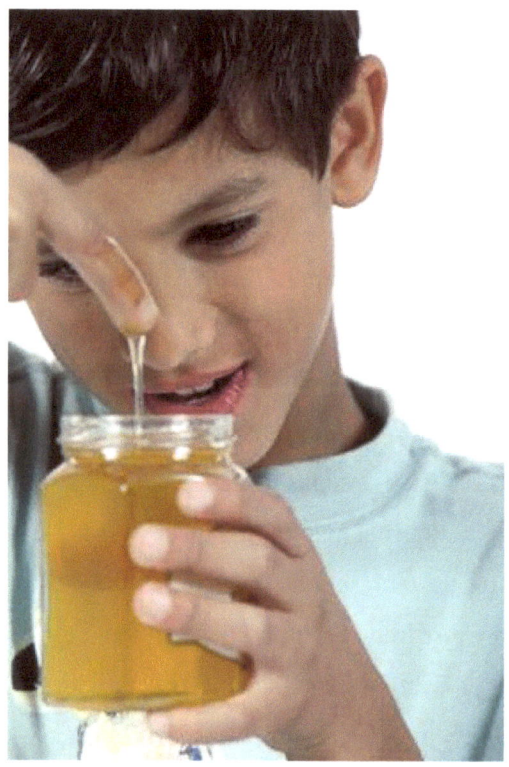

But remember, lots of vinegar, taken in lots of quantities can have an adverse affect on your teeth, especially when your teeth begin to get sensitive. If you are using vinegar as a mouth rinse, make sure that it does not stay long in your mouth. Do not swirl it around continuously, when you are using it as a gargle or a mouthwash. After you have spat out the vinegar, remove all vestiges of it by a baking soda solution, to counteract the acidic content. Also, using vinegar in large quantities over a long period of time is going to have the same debilitating effect upon your bones, well, elementary my dear Watson, if it can have this effect on your teeth made up of calcium, wanted to have the same on your bones, thus causing osteoporosis?

If you are using vinegar as a cleansing agent, remember to dilute it with water, especially when you are using it on smooth surfaces like glass and metal.

Even today, I see my mother using malt vinegar on newspaper to give that extra gloss to glass windows. She learned that as a girl in England in 1954, and I think this way to clear mirrors and windows which are smeared with dirt, grime, and grease is quite effective. I went one step further and used this newspaper/malt vinegar idea for cleaning my glass and stainless steel containers, as a last polish. Not much elbow grease required here, which you would need to expend when you are polishing glasses with just an ordinary cloth. Also, she learned in war-torn Europe that the best way to clean any food items like fruit and vegetables was by putting them in salt and vinegar water before cooking to get rid of the bacteria, fungi, and other harmful organisms.

Also, a good housekeeping magazine of that particular period had this helpful household hint. When you want to get rid of the wallpaper and do not know how to get the glue off, just coat with a mixture of boiling hot water to which you have added 5 tablespoons full of vinegar. Keep it on, and then you shall see that wallpaper just peeling off like an onion skin.

Well, dear Watson, boiling hot water on paper, left on, duh; of course it would remove wallpaper. But the vinegar gets rid of the glue. So that is all right.

Making a Vinegar Tincture

A tincture is normally made up of herbs preserved in alcohol. In ancient times, these herbs were preserved in wine by boiling them in the wine, so that all the good essential oils and the beneficial qualities of that particular Herb could be infused in the boiled wine.

If you look at any old herbal book, where you are looking for a recipe for a tincture, you are going to see – without any full stops, take just a handful of this particular herb or a handful of that particular herb and then boil in a barrel full of wine until you get the color and then "drink freely of it".

Well, where are the barrel full of wines so easily available in your cellar today. Who has those huge cooking spaces in the kitchens, where you could boil a whole barrel full of wine, with plenty of herbs? Nevertheless, you can make your own tinctures with fresh and dried ingredients. Some of the herbs are going to need different strengths of alcohol 15 – 90% proof, and in Russia, vodka is still the excellent traditional base for tinctures. A standard ratio is going to be 25 g of dried herb or 50 g of fresh herb to every 2 ½ cups of alcoholic liquid. Well. That is better. This looks manageable!

This is the same proportion which you are going to use when you are using vinegar as a tincture base. These are going to keep indefinitely and the dosage is very small, yet it is very effective. If you are giving this to a child, remember to put the dose in half a cup of water and leave uncovered for a number of hours until all the alcoholic content has evaporated. This is of course only if you have made your tincture in alcoholic bases like wine or vodka. But if it is the vinegar-based tincture, even then you can put 5 drops in 4 tablespoons full of water to dilute the acetic content, especially when you are giving it to a little youngster.

Traditional spiced wine or spiced vinegar is excellent for catching the true flavor of herbs when they are diluted with water or fruit juices, and served iced or cold. For example, you can make a pleasant spiced wine by taking a favorite wine like a light white wine or a rose and adding a fresh sprig of rosemary, 4 cardamom seeds, 4 cloves, and just a twist of lemon peel to the mixture and allowing it to steep for as long as you like. You can either drink it fresh or you can drink it after a couple of days.

A tincture tonic is normally taken from anywhere between 5 drops to one teaspoonful once a day. A standard treatment is taking 1 teaspoon, 3 times a day. For an acute condition take 1 teaspoon, 6 times a day. Diluted tincture is going to be made up of 1 teaspoon to 1 cup water to make a wash, gargle, or a compress.

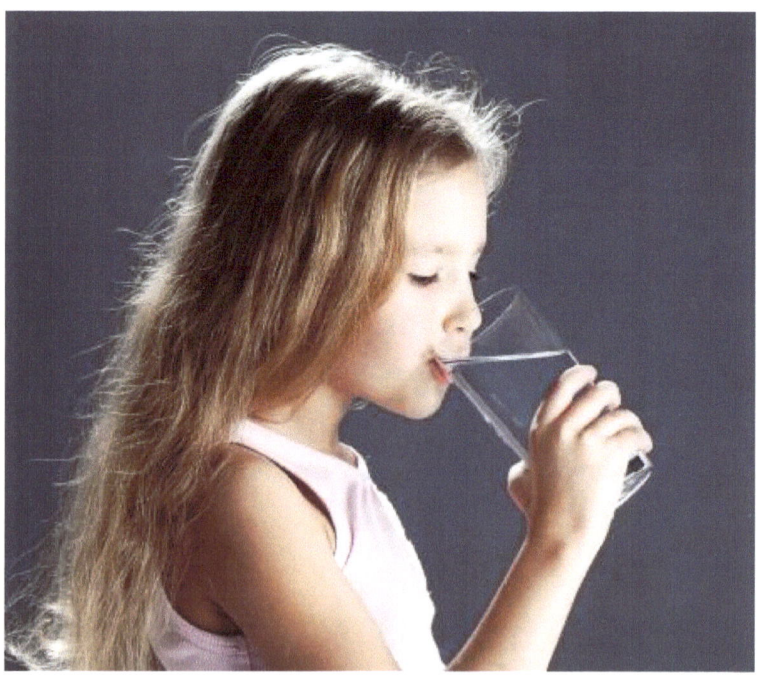

Dilute a bit of tincture in water, if you have made it with an alcohol base. Then allow the water to remain for a number of hours in the open air, so that the alcohol content disappears.

Make up your vinegar tincture by taking 7/8 th – 200 mL – cup vinegar, 15 g dried herbs (25 g fresh herbs), and 6 tablespoons full of water. This is going to make 1 ¾ cups.

Scissor and bruise the herbs, so that you can get all the essential oils out of the leaves and stems. Mix the vinegar together along with the water. Put the herbs into a large jar and add the liquid – if you do not want to make this tincture out of vinegar, you can also make it out of any sort of spirit like brandy or vodka – 200 mL – 7/8 cup – and after that, put it in a cool dark place for the next 2 weeks. Remember to shake and turn upside down daily.

After 2 weeks, the liquid will have absorbed all the natural goodness of the herbs and the color of the liquid will have changed. You may think it tempting to leave the mixture to stand a little bit longer. **Do not do that.** After one certain point this extra material is not going to strengthen the mixture and the herb is going to break down chemically.

Strain through a loose weave cotton cloth placed over a container, squeeze and ring the herbs in the glass to get out every drop of the precious liquid. This is your tincture. The herbs can be used for cooking. Pour the strained liquid into clean glass bottles. Amber is best because it is dark.

Tonic herbs taken in their infused form were normally taken by our ancestors over a long period of time with 25 g of herbs and 50 g of spices to every 7 1/2 cups of red or white wine or alcoholic liquid made with 2 parts of spirits to one part of water. This tonic wine and spirit was made the same way you made your herbal tincture in vinegar/spirits. ¼ cup was taken twice a day. Do not take more than 2 times are more than 50 mL and you can dilute with warm water, if you think that the alcoholic content is really strong.

I saw a friend of mine taking this wine tonic as an aperitif 20 minutes before eating, because according to him, it stimulated the appetite. And then he ate and he ate. Well, he was used to that since his twenties!

Vinegar and Brown Paper Poultice

When Jill came down the hill, running back home as fast as she could caper, Jack went to bed to mend his head with vinegar and brown paper. Incidentally, this nursery rhyme has something of sense in it, where you can use vinegar and brown paper as a poultice.

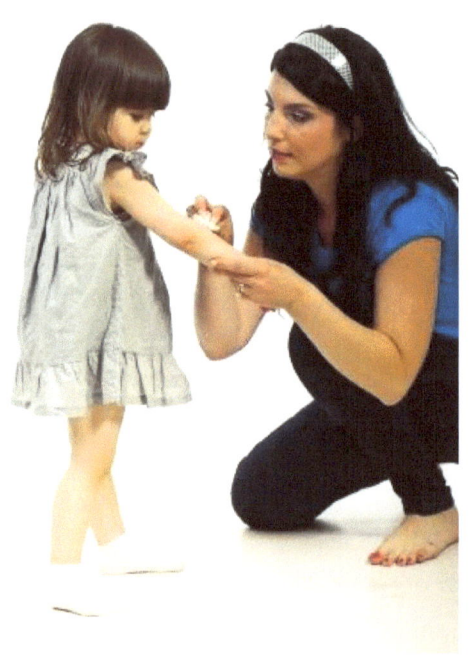

It was used extensively in Victorian times and all you have to do is take 5/6 sheets of strong brown paper in a pan and cover with vinegar. But before that, that particular vinegar is going to be infused with an herb to cool and reduce the swelling and bring the bruises to the surface. The herb which we use here is sage.

These are traditional ingredients, often used in compresses, and in poultices. Any sort of sprain, and vinegar and brown paper poultice, and you are going to find yourself healing really fast.

You are first going to bruise fresh sage leaves. You can use a flat surface, place the leaves and then roll over them with your rolling pin. Do not tear them or break them. Now put the Sage leaves in a pan and just covered with vinegar. Simmer gently for 5 minutes over a very low heat. The vinegar should not boil but it should steam so that the Sage leaves blanch, soften, and infuse the vinegar with their natural healing ingredients.

After 5 minutes, take out the leaves and lay them down on a cloth. Work quickly and carefully as the leaves are still very hot. Fold the cloth into a package that just covers the affected area. This is of course a vinegar and sage poultice. Apply as hard as you can bear it and cover with towels to retain the heat. Leave on for an hour and see the swelling subsiding.

You can also dilute the vinegar with warm water and use it as a fomentation for bruises and sprains. When it is diluted with iced water, it is going to make an excellent compress for hot and swollen joints and also for hot tension headaches.

For vinegar and brown paper, the paper was covered with sage vinegar in a container, a lid put on it and steamed over a very low heat for a few minutes.

This is going to depend on the type of paper. It needs to soften and absorb the vinegar without disintegrating or tearing into pieces.

Take out the paper; wrap it up in overlapping layers around the affected part. Cover all the areas as hot as possible because this is some sort of fomentation with the vinegar. You will need to build up several layers. Cover with plastic or cling film to keep the heat in and bandage. Leave on for 4 hours. Reapply twice a day until the swelling and bruising has subsided. A hot vinegar fomentation feels very strengthening, supportive, and grateful.

A friend of mine told me that she took Apple cider vinegar and bicarbonate soda for acid reflux, but I would not advise taking it regularly, because it is preventing your natural healing system in your body to work in an unnatural way with the influx of something acidic and something basic to counteract it. Instead, watch your diet, and instead try yogurt with honey to cure your system. Stop eating spicy and fatty food for a couple of weeks to see how much the reflux has improved with the addition of healthy bacteria to your stomach. Also, forget about cola drinks, tea, and coffee.

Cannot do without tea, you say? Try a soothing herbal tea made up of sage leaves with a touch of cinnamon to heal your stomach. If you are a coffee addict and cannot do without caffeine, try chewing pieces of licorice with rock candy and honey instead. They are going to give you enough liquid in your mouth to get rid of that caffeine craving. Also, they are going to heal your stomach.

Vinegar As a Beauty Product

Vinegar because of its acid content is excellent as a beauty product, especially for the hair and ancient beauties did not hesitate in rinsing their hair with beer and vinegar, after washing it.

Vinegar Hair Rinse

A vinegar hair rinse is going to keep the scalp healthy, and the hair conditioned well. Dilute one tablespoonful of herbal vinegar with 250 mL or 1 cup of water. Rub thoroughly into the hair and scalp. Leave on for 5 minutes and then rinse off. If you have dark hair, you are going to use sage to darken it. Lemon and chamomile are used to lighten the hair. Parsley is excellent for curing dandruff conditions and rosemary is good for conditioning brittle, falling, and dry hair.

Using Vinegar for Anti-aging.

We are going to be using pure apple cider vinegar here. Make up a mixture of 3 teaspoons full of Apple cider vinegar, 2 teaspoons full of honey, half a cup each of almond oil, glycerin and Rosewater. Add one teaspoonful of lemon juice to this mixture. Bottle it, and before you go to sleep, you are going to wash your face clean with hot water without using any soap. Now just dip a ball of cotton in this mixture, just enough to clean your neck, and face. After you have got all the vestiges of grime out, just take a little bit of this mixture in the palm of your hand and apply it all over your face and neck. Allow just enough time for the almond oil to get absorbed, before you get into bed, otherwise you are going to be complaining of oil stains on the pillows!

Believe it or not, this is one way in which you will never suffer from wrinkles or lines, even when you are in your seventies or eighties. I started this in my twenties, from a recipe given to me by one of my friends just to get rid of the grime after a day spent in a pollution soaked teeming metropolis, – wear your white uniform outside and reach your office, 20 minutes later with a grimy gray sooty speckled uniform; we soon learned to carry our formal white and navy blue uniforms with us and change them in the office lunch and relaxation rooms, having reached it in a T-shirt and jeans which could be as grimy as ever traveling outside because they would not be seen by the general public. And soon I found out that my skin looked better and younger and best of all, I had never suffered from any sort of wrinkles and skin problems as the decades went by.

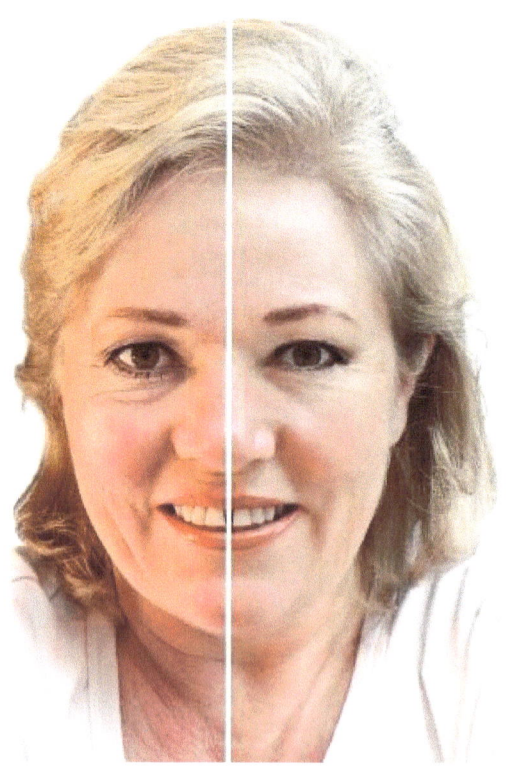

I think it is because of the vinegar and honey which are excellent antiseptic and antioxidant agents. Try it out.

Conclusion

This book has introduced you to vinegar and how it has been used down the centuries to help heal you and also to keep you beautiful. So make up your own vinegar tinctures, and vinegar tonics and keep healthy.

Piccallilli

So there I was, some pages ago, talking about Piccallilli, – which is pickles gone very wrong indeed, with apologies to Rudyard Kipling – but here is the recipe. For this, you are going to use one large cauliflower broken up into 1 inch florets, 2 cucumbers, cut into cubes of half an inch, 2 pounds of shallots and onions, diced and sliced, 2 pounds of apples, your favorite sort, cut into half an inch cubes, 4.5 L of water in which you have dissolved 450 g of salt, 25 g of chili peppers, 50 g of garlic cloves, 25 g of root ginger crashed, 25 g of black peppercorns, 2.2 L of vinegar – 10 cups, 50 g of cornstarch or corn flour, 1 ounce [25 g] of turmeric, this is going to be ground fresh after you have roasted the corm to fix the color. Turmeric is necessary because after all, the origins were Eastern and nothing can do without a golden color, and 1 ounce of mustard powder, for the spicy, pungent, piquant mustard taste.

Cover the vegetables and the fruit with cold brine and let stand overnight. After that, drain and pack into hot sterilized jars. Brine the whole spices in vinegar for 5 minutes. Blend the cornstarch, turmeric, and mustard with a little bit of cold vinegar and then stir into the boiling vinegar. Boil for 10 minutes more.

Pour over the vegetables, filling the jars and seal once it is cool. Store in a cool, dark place. This is going to take about 6 weeks in order to give its full flavor. This is going to keep indefinitely. But once you have opened it, you will need to refrigerate it.

This, of course, is not the original traditional recipe, with mustard powder being used as a substitute for pure mustard oil in which the vegetables were preserved, instead of being preserved in brine. The true pickles are going to have lots and lots of extra spices and lots of hot chilies, fried beforehand in mustard seeds and mustard oil and then all the vegetables are going to be thrown into them, and cooked.

After that, the preserving is done in mustard oil and salt instead of salt brine.

I have some traditional pickles going back to 10 years or more and all I do is top them off once every 2 years with hot mustard oil, and they take on a new lease of life. But then I have this bad habit of eating the mustard oil, with all its spice and flavor, which is nice and spicy instead of eating the pickles and one fine day, I find my glass pickle jars nearly dry without any oil in them!

Also, when talking about which herb went well, with which particular vinegar, I spoke about apple mint.

So this is how you are going to make apple mint vinegar – not the fermented variety, where you are going to be using mint – mint according to taste – and apple peels in vinegar – and really quickly.

Apple Mint Vinegar

250 mL – 1 cup of apple juice a pinch of ground cinnamon, one tablespoonful of apple cider vinegar, and half a cup full of chopped mint.

Mix the ingredients together and pour into a glass containing ice. Dilute according to taste with water.

Live Long and Prosper!

Author Bio

Dueep Jyot Singh is a Management and IT Professional who managed to gather Postgraduate qualifications in Management and English and Degrees in Science, French and Education while pursuing different enjoyable career options like being an hospital administrator, IT,SEO and HRD Database Manager/ trainer, movie , radio and TV scriptwriter, theatre artiste and public speaker, lecturer in French, Marketing and Advertising, ex-Editor of Hearts On Fire (now known as Solstice) Books Missouri USA, advice columnist and cartoonist, publisher and Aviation School trainer, ex-moderator on Medico.in, banker, student councilor ,travelogue writer … among other things!

One fine morning, she decided that she had enough of killing herself by Degrees and went back to her first love—writing. It's more enjoyable! She already has 48 published academic and 14 fiction- in- different- genre books under her belt.

When she is not designing websites or making Graphic design illustrations for clients , she is browsing through old bookshops hunting for treasures, of which she has an enviable collection – including R.L. Stevenson, O.Henry, Dornford Yates, Maurice Walsh, De Maupassant, Victor Hugo, Sapper, C.N. Williamson, "Bartimeus" and the crown of her collection- Dickens "The Old Curiosity Shop," and "Martin Chuzzlewit" and so on… Just call her "Renaissance Woman" - collecting herbal remedies, acting like Universal Helping Hand/Agony Aunt, or escaping to her dear mountains for a bit of exploring, collecting herbs and plants, and trekking.

Check out some of the other JD-Biz Publishing books

Gardening Series on Amazon

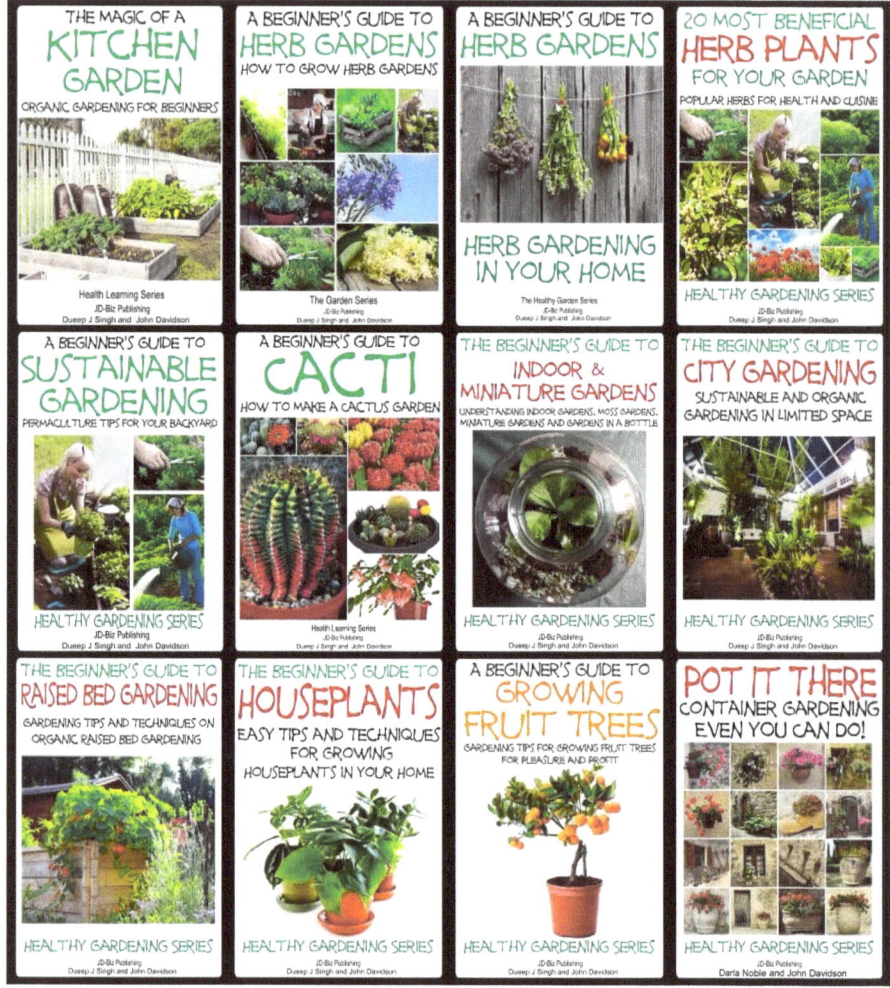

Download Free Books!

http://MendonCottageBooks.com

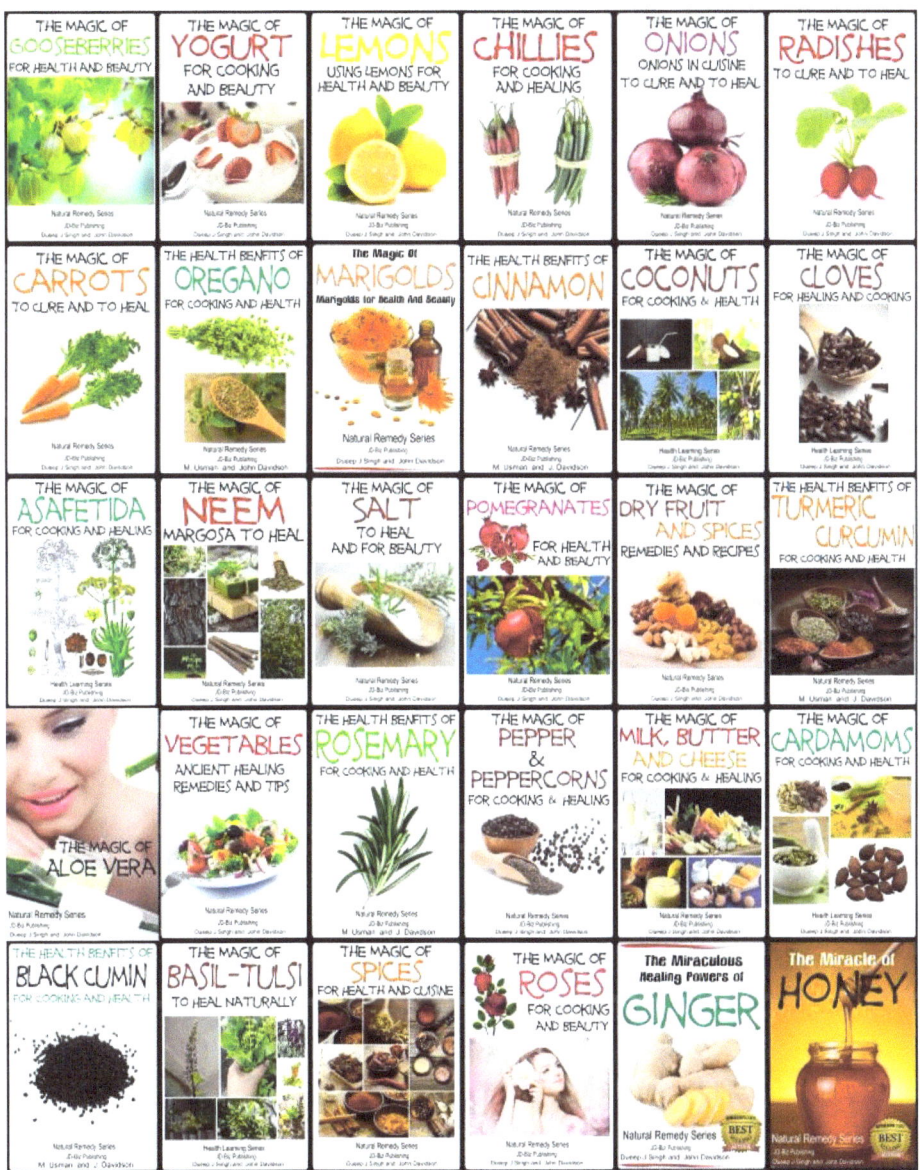

Country Life Books

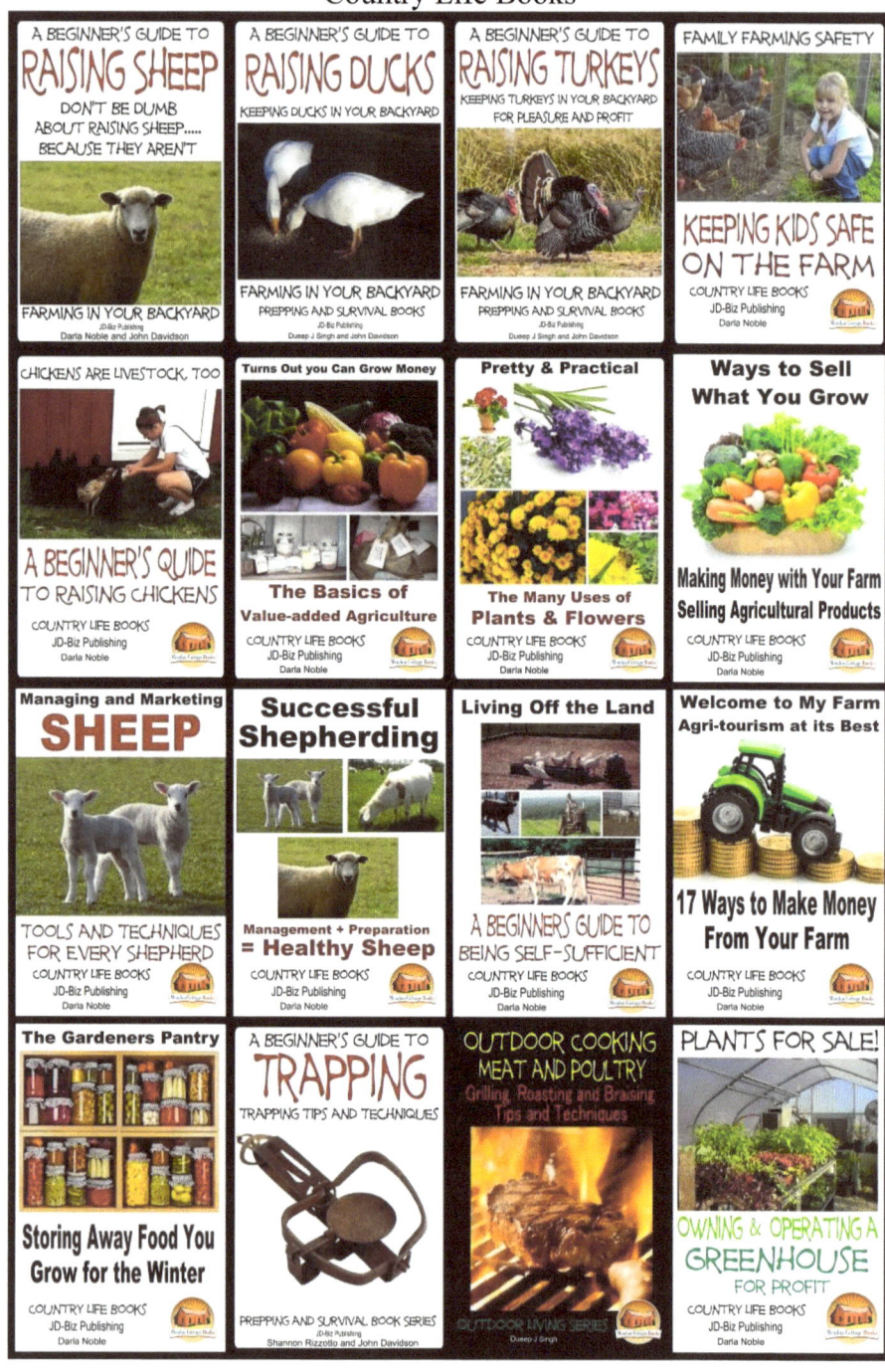

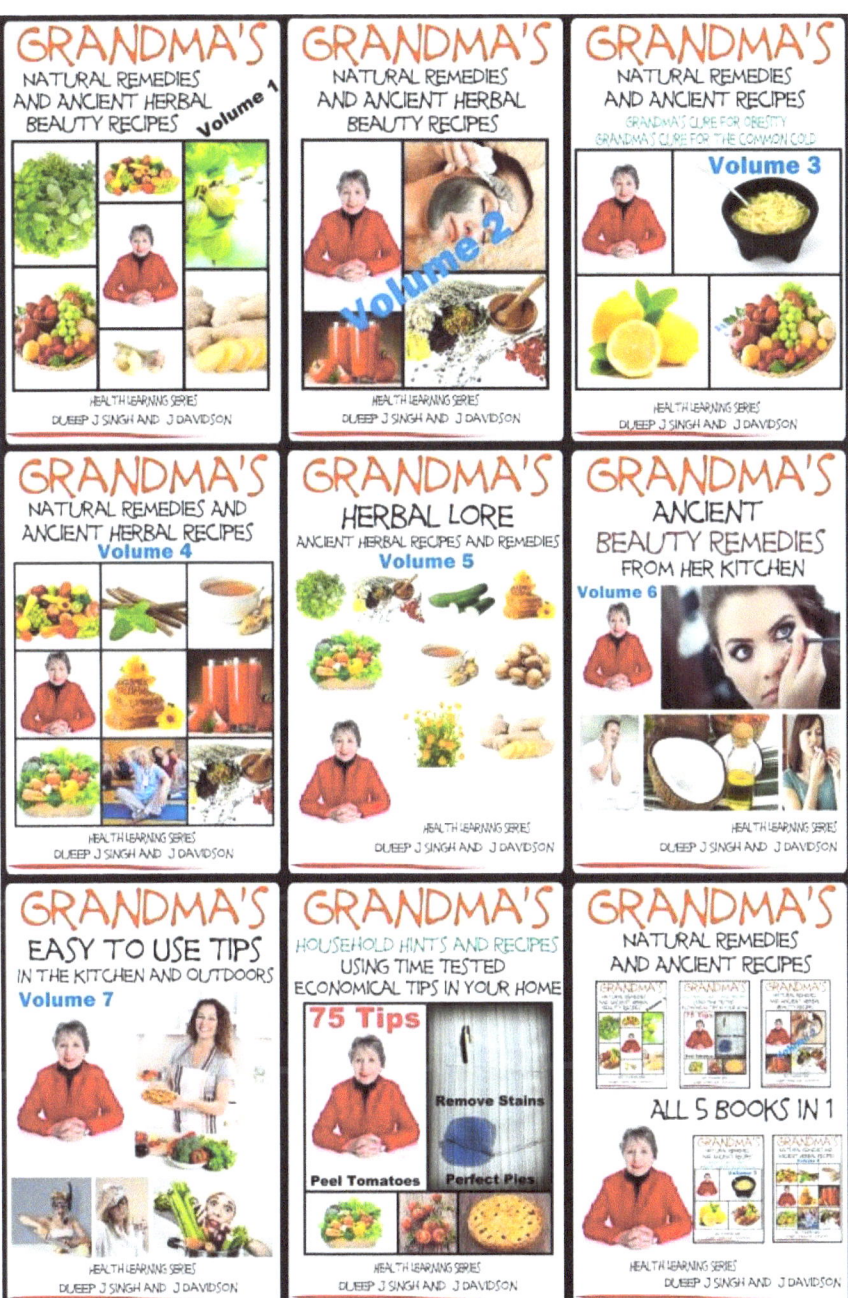

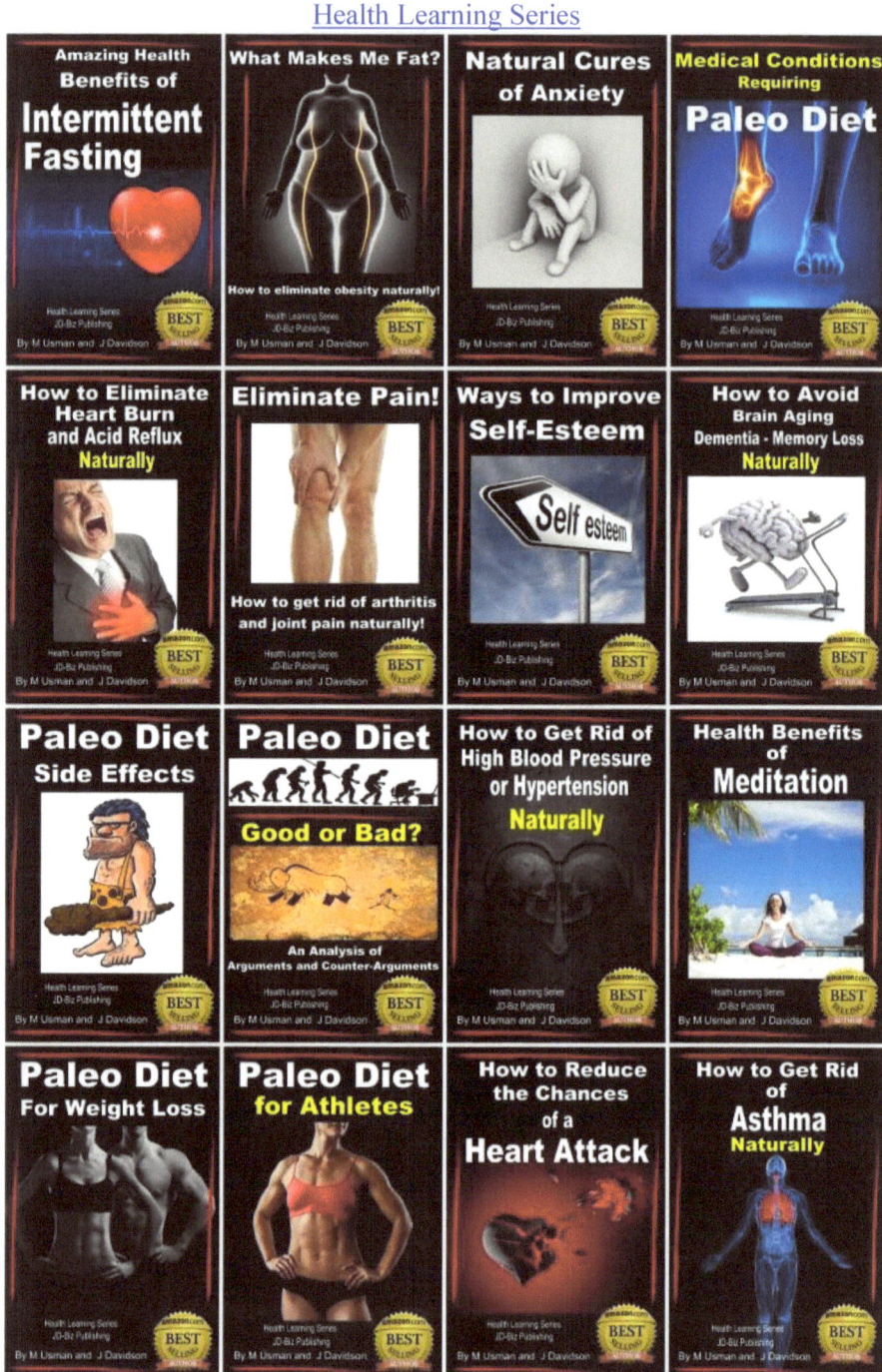

Amazing Animal Book Series

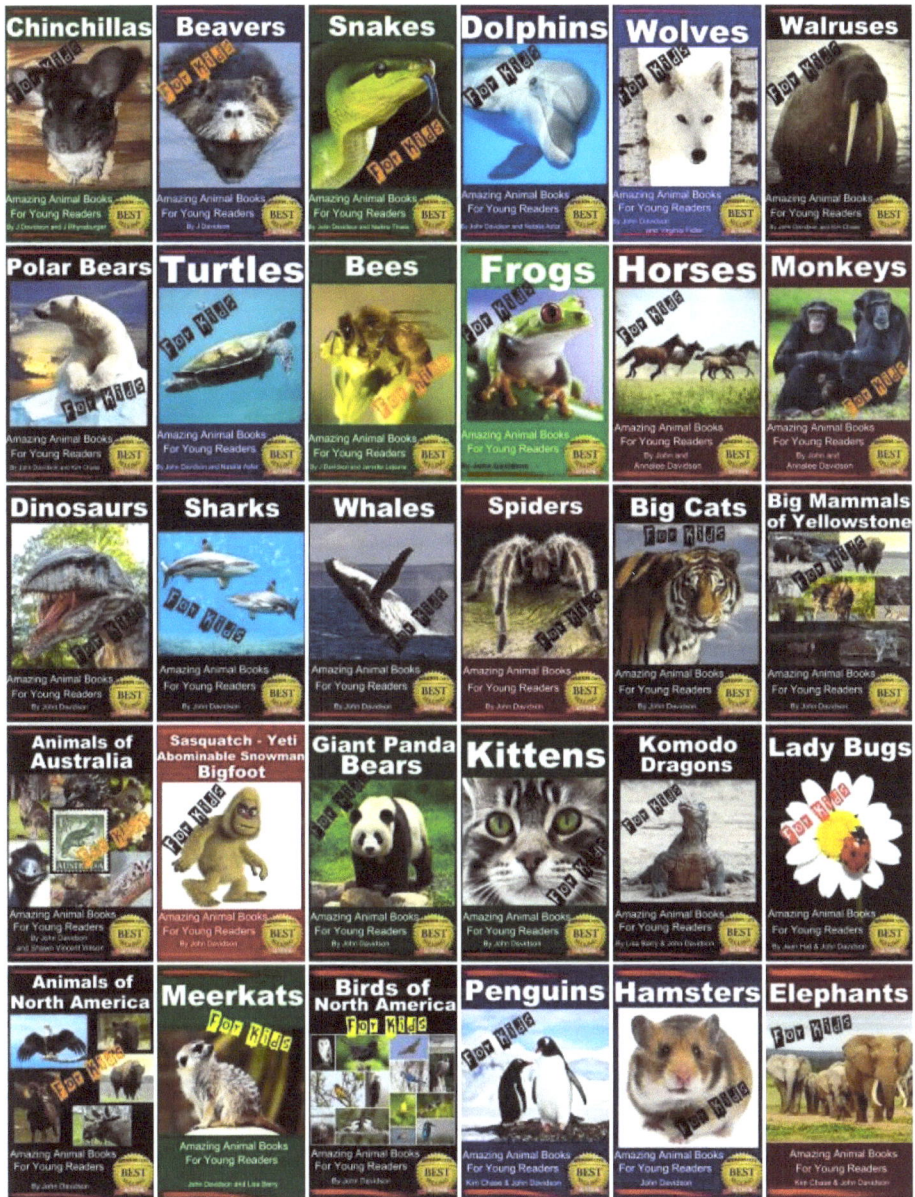

Learn To Draw Series

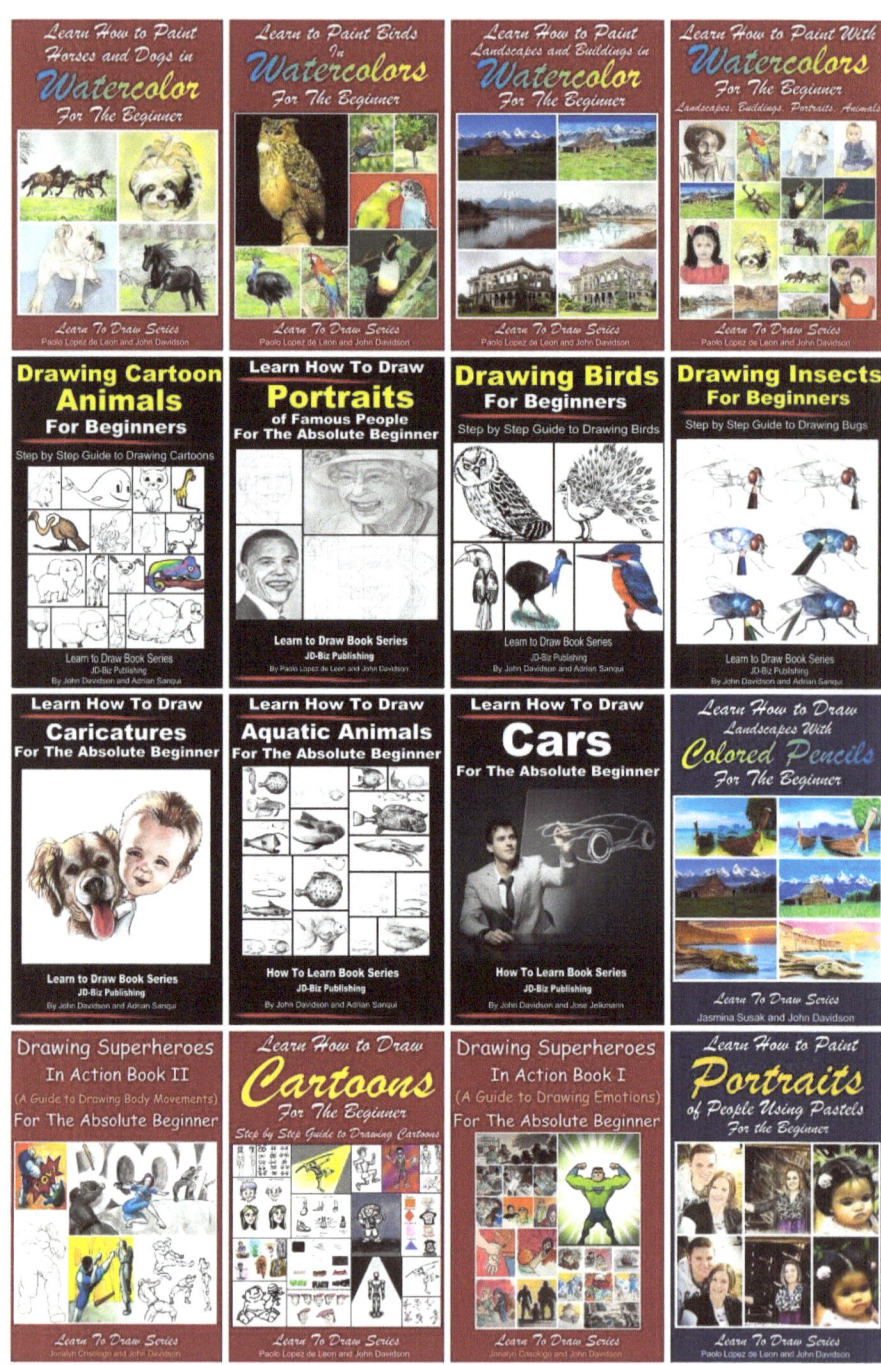

How to Build and Plan Books

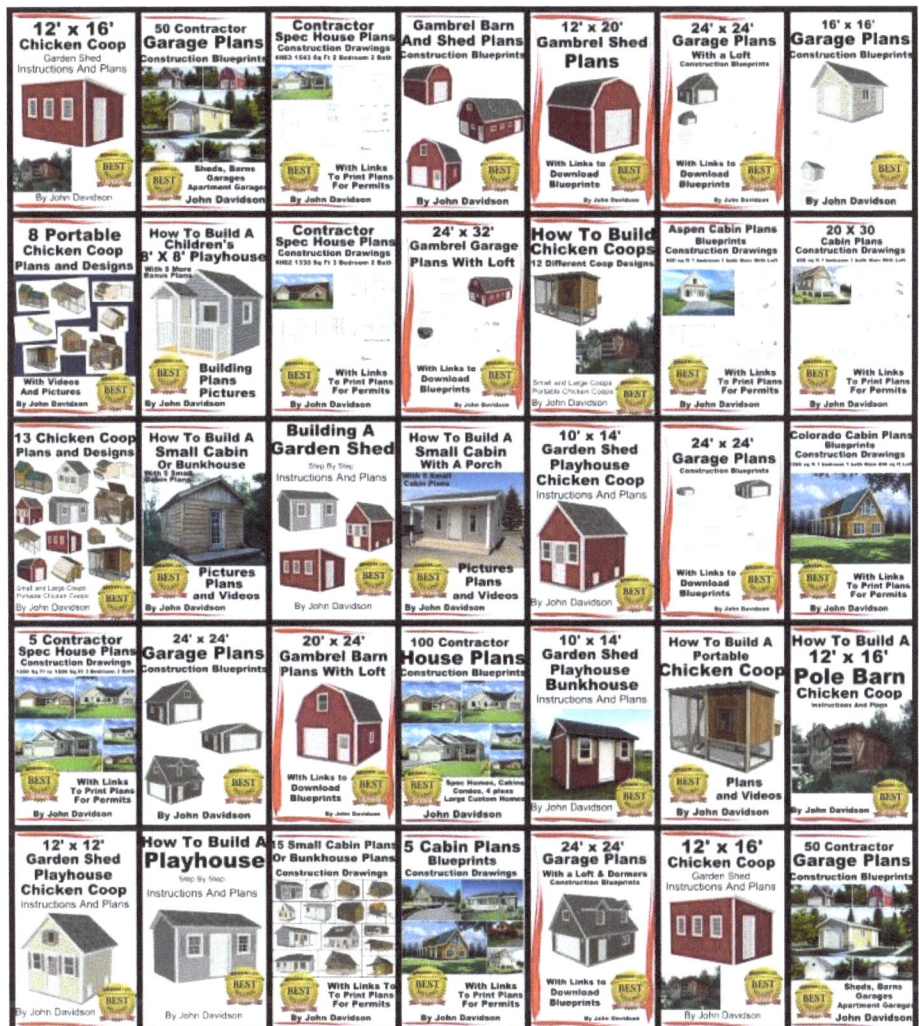

Entrepreneur Book Series

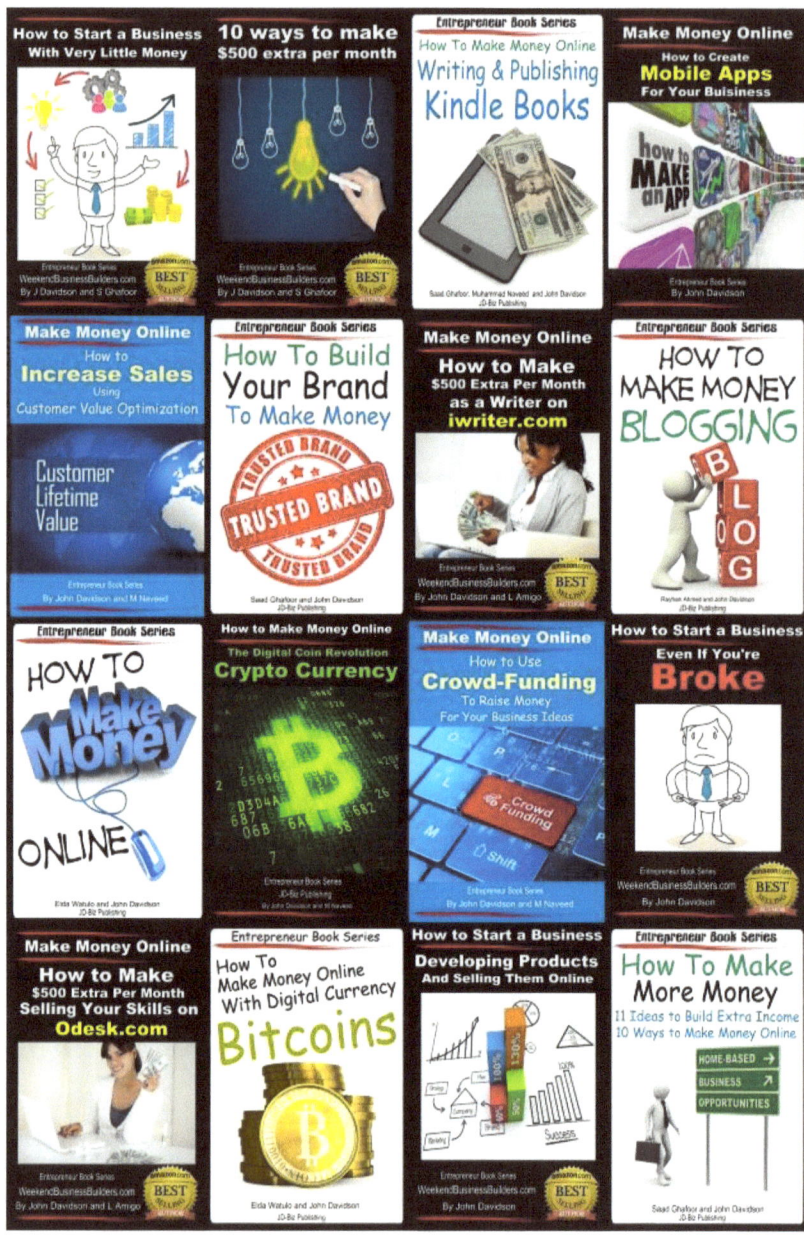

Our books are available at

1. Amazon.com

2. Barnes and Noble

3. Itunes

4. Kobo

5. Smashwords

6. Google Play Books

Download Free Books!

http://MendonCottageBooks.com

Publisher

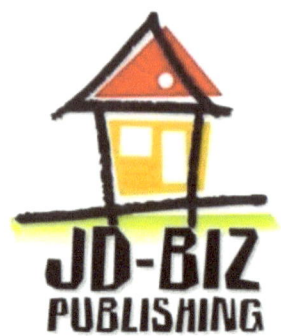

JD-Biz Corp

P O Box 374

Mendon, Utah 84325

http://www.jd-biz.com/

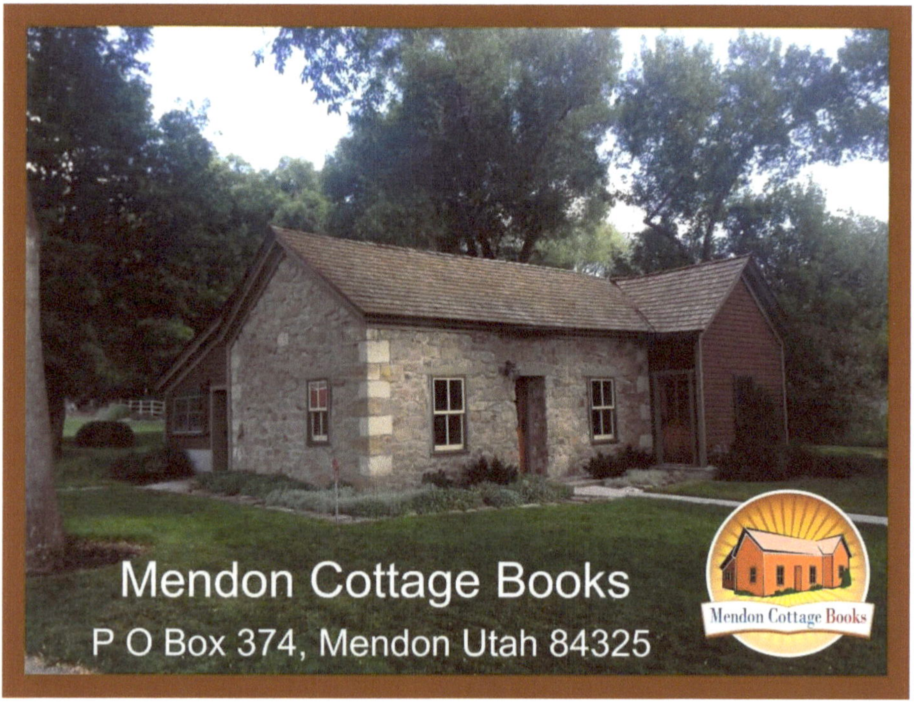

Mendon Cottage Books

P O Box 374, Mendon Utah 84325

Mendon Cottage Books

www.ingramcontent.com/pod-product-compliance
Lightning Source LLC
Chambersburg PA
CBHW050820290526
45792CB00001B/197